PHYSICAL VASCULAR THERAPY - THE NEXT GENERATION OF MEDICINE?

MICROCIRCULATION OF BLOOD - WHAT EVERYONE SHOULD KNOW ABOUT

PETER CARL SIMONS

ISBN 978-1-63920-244-7

Contents

Acknowledgements

Bemer Products are made by Bemer International AG in Triesen, Liechtenstein

Prologue

The human body relies heavily on blood and other fluids that flow through the blood vessels. From veins to arteries and their smaller versions, the body has a lot of vessels transporting nutrients to organs and removing waste materials from the same organs. While the bigger vessels in the body can be easily dealt with using simple operations, the very small capillaries, venules, and arterioles cannot be operated upon with physical equipment. For this reason, major companies such as the Bemer Group have invested heavily in the aspects of their treatment to help people with problems at the microscopic levels of their blood circulation. For the most part, their research has led them to the science of physical vascular therapy. This science has developed over time and has become a mainstream aspect of medical treatment today. The focus of this treatment is to make it possible to carry out diagnosis and treatment of problems of the circulatory system that cannot be solved in any other way. For this case, we will focus on the physical vascular therapy technology provided by Bemer which is the leading firm in this field. But, first of all, let us delve into defining microcirculation and how physical vascular therapy promotes it to have better circulation in the rest of the body.

ONE
MICROCIRCULATION

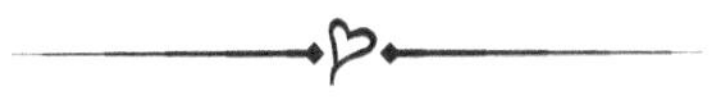

The microcirculation of blood has been defined in several ways although the common agreement is the movement of blood in the smallest blood vessels of the body. These blood vessels are found in the section of the body called the vasculature that is embedded in the tissues of the body.

It may get confusing when one hears of microcirculation and macrocirculation. As stated before, microcirculation is used in reference to the circulation of blood within organs and with the small blood vessels. On the other hand, microcirculation occurs between organs the veins we see on our hands are part of the microcirculation system. You cannot see microcirculation with the naked eye given that it is made up of capillaries, arterioles, and venules which are too small for the eye to see. These small vessels work by draining capillary blood from the main vessels and the organs of the body. When visualizing how the process of microcirculation works, one can see that blood will flow from the heart to the arteries towards the organs. Upon reaching the organs, the blood arteries branch out into arterioles which are smaller than the arteries themselves. The arterioles further branch out to the capillaries which are the smallest of blood vessels.

It is through the walls of the capillaries that materials are exchanged between the blood and the organs of the body. After the exchange, the blood will flow from the capillaries which combine to form the venules. The venules further combine to form the veins which take blood back to the heart and lungs for purification and pumping.

Arterioles

Arterioles are the branches of the arteries which carry blood to the organs. When arteries reach the organs and tissues of the body, they branch out to create the arterioles. These blood vessels are innervated meaning they are supplied with nerves all around. The vessels are also surrounded by smooth muscle cells. The arterioles carry blood from the arteries to the capillaries which are even smaller than the arterioles. Their diameter is between 10 to 100 µm.

Capillaries

The capillaries are branches of the arterioles. They lack smooth muscle cells around them, unlike the arterioles. They also lack nerves around them hence are not inner gated. Their diameter ranges from. 5 to 8 µm. Due to the lack of smooth muscle cells and nerves, the capillaries have thinner walls than any other blood vessel in the body. They thus permeate easy movement of materials from them to the rest of the body tissue or from the tissue to the bloodstream.

Venules

Of the three small blood vessels, the venues are the largest. Their diameter ranges from 10 to 200 µm. Although they still have smooth muscles around them, they are fewer than their found in arterioles. From the capillaries, blood will flow out to the venules which combine to form the veins that are visible to the naked eye.

Other Vessels

Besides the arterioles, capillaries and venules, there are vessels of the body that are also involved in the process of microcirculation such as lymphatic capillaries and collecting ducts.

The focus of microcirculation is to deliver oxygen and nutrients to the body tissues while removing wastes such as carbon dioxide from them. Given that the process of microcirculation regulates the flow of blood and the perfusion of tissues, it has a direct effect on the pressure of blood in the body. The pericyte cells are responsible for the regulation of the pressure of blood at the microcirculation level since they can expand and contract thus varying the size of the diameter of the arterioles. In this way, the pressure of blood flowing through the tissues is determined in the arterioles as it enters the tissues. The process of responding to inflammation with results such as edema and swelling is similar to this one in every aspect.

A look at the vessels that carry out microcirculation reveals a structure that is made up of the endothelium cells which have a flattened structure. Most of the endothelium cells are surrounded by pericyte cells which have contractile properties. The structure of the endothelium makes it the best for the flow of blood in the tissues and vessels of the body. Another advantage it has it that it allows for the easy and quick movement of the water and dissolved minerals from the blood found in the interstitial plasma and the tissues of the body. The endothelium also has the task of producing the molecules which act by preventing blood clotting in the tissues. If the blood clotted in this small vessels, it would be easy to prevent the actual flow of blood in the whole tissue. These molecules stop their work the moment they sense a leak of blood. They allow clotting as it will preserve the life of the organism.

TWO
SECTORS OF MICROCIRCULATION

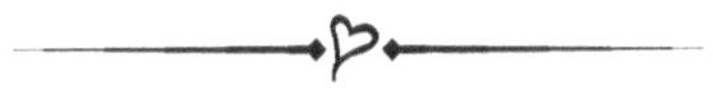

Blood at the microcirculation level operates in stages which are called sectors. There are three sectors of the microcirculation from the pre-capillary (resistive) sector, the capillary (swap) sector, and the post-capillary (capacitive) sector.

Pre-capillary sector

Before blood goes into the venules and capillaries, the arteriole and pre-capillary sphincter sworn by regulating the pressure and generals flow of the blood. Due to the presence of the smooth muscles that are embedded in the walls of the venules and arterioles, they are able to contract and relax to increase and reduce the pressure of the blood respectively.

Capillary sector

This is the most vital of the three sectors. This sector involves the blood flowing through the capillaries. This flow of blood allows the exchange of substances such as gasses, dissolved minerals, and others to and from the interstitial fluid in the body tissues and the bloodstream. The substances that move from the bloodstream into the interstitial fluid are mainly nutrients and oxygen while the substances that move across the walls of the capillaries are the wastes such as carbon dioxide. These exchanges occur through the walls of the capillaries suing certain processes we shall dwell on later.

Post-capillary sector

The exchange of substances does not end with the capillary sector. In the post-capillary sector, there is still a movement of substances across the walls of the blood vessels also to a smaller scale than in the capillary sector. The blood vessels involved are called the post-capillary venules and are made up of a layer of endothelial cells. After the final exchange of substances, the blood leaves the organ to the veins.

The Regulation of Microcirculation

This process of microcirculation, although it occurs at a microscopic level of the body, it requires a high level of regulation to keep the whole body working as designed. This is due to the fact that this level of circulation determines what happens to the blood in the rest of the body. The first process involved at this level of circulation is that if tissue perfusion. The relaxing and contracting of the walls of the arterioles serves as a control mechanism for the blood flowing through the capillaries. The vascular diameter and tone of the blood vessels are determined by the relaxing and contracting of the walls of the arterioles. These contractions and relaxations are in response to the various stimuli types that activate the vascular smooth muscles. An example would be when there is the distending of the blood vessels. In this case, the level of pressure of the blood flowing through the tissues would be increased. This aspect serves as stimuli for the arterial wall muscles. To keep the pressure within the normal parameters, the arterial wall muscles will contract and thus keep the blood pressure in the normal parameters. If the inverse happens, there is another step that will be observed. If the blood vessels in the body contract and increase the level of pressure in the body, the arteriolar wall muscles respond by relaxing and allowing more blood to flow into the tissue. The amount of blood allowed in is just within the parameters of the norm. This aspect ensures that the blood pressure in the body tissues remains at a constant level even if the pressure in the rest of body is fluctuating from the safe limits. The pressure of the blood within the tissues has to remain within this given limits since this level of pressure is the best for the exchange of materials between the tissues and the blood. Too much pressure and the exchange will not occur while there is too low pressure will also not allow an exchange given there would be no difference in the concentration of substances between the fluid in the cells and the blood.

The microcirculation process is also controlled by the nervous system of the body. The first part of the nervous system that controls the microcirculation system is the sympathetic nervous system. It works by activating the smaller terminals and arterioles. Besides that, the nervous system releases certain compounds that make it possible to regulate the microcirculation system further. They include neuropeptides, neurotransmitters, and hormones like catecholamine, remind-angiotensin, vasopressin, atrial natriuretic peptide, noradrenaline, adrenaline and many others. These hormones will affect the microcirculation system in different ways and in accordance with the prevailing conditions. However, their effects can be can be clarified to value two main scenarios namely vasoconstriction and vasodilation. They also have effects on the beta and alpha adrenergic receptors.

It is actually a complex process when one looks at the working of the arterioles and the other small vessels of the body. Their working is largely determined by the presence and absence of metabolic stimuli which are generated or secreted from various parts of the body. For the arterioles to vasodilate, the level of catabolic Proust in the tissues has to be considerably high for the vasodilation to be triggered. The level of metabolism determines the level of catabolic products in the tissues in the tissues. The higher the metabolism level, the higher the catabolic products. Through vasodilation, the endothelium can have control on the muscle cells' tone and the flow of blood in the arterioles. Besides that, the endothelium can circulate, activate and inactivate any substances in the plasma like the hormones. The endothelium controls the blood vessels' diameter within the tissues through the secretion of many substances which end up acting as vasoconstrictors and vasodilators. What one can learn from this is that all the channels in the blood vessels located in the tissues in the body are as a result of the responses in the body to the conditions prevailing in the body.

The Process of Microcirculatory Exchange

This process of microcirculatory exchange, popularly called the capillary exchange process, is the process of exchanging substances across the walls of the capillaries of the body. Given that capillaries are the result of the branching out first of the arteries to form arterioles then further branching to form them, they are the highest in number and also the smallest in size. This high number and small size is meant to cover as much of the tissue as possible. Their Hugh numbers and small sizes are also focused on reducing the distance that the substances diffusing across their walls into and out of the body tissues would cover to make the tissues healthy. They have very thin walls that do not have either muscles or nerves as these would increase the thickness of their walls. This thinness is meant to increase the surface area on which the exchange occurs between the blood and the tissues. Also, the thin walls considerably reduce the distance traveled by the substances entering and leaving the bloodstream and the tissues. At any one time of an individual, 7 percent of the total blood in the body is contained in the capillaries. That is where the exchange of materials between the interstitial fluid and the blood takes place. The name capillary exchange is given to this exchange process that occurs between the blood and the interstitial fluid.

The capillary exchange takes place in three main processes namely diffusion, bulk flow and transcytosis (vesicular transport). The exchange in solids, liquids and even gasses between the blood and interstitial fluid involves post-capillaries, collecting venules and capillary venules. All the activities of the capillary exchange process take place here but for the plasma proteins. The plasma proteins, being too big, cannot go through the walls. After the first pass of the blood in the capillaries fails to absorb the large particles such as the plasma proteins, there is a second pass in which the molecules' kinetic motion is used to absorb them into the interstitial fluid in the tissues.

THREE

THE REGULATION OF CAPILLARY EXCHANGE

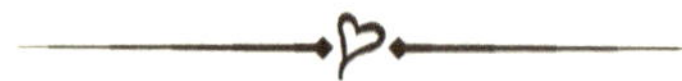

There are many mechanisms which go into the regulating the process of microcirculation. All these mechanisms work alongside each other and make it possible for the quick, efficient and complete exchange of materials.

Diffusion

Given that the rate of diffusion is inversely related to the distance between the cells and the capillaries, the rate of diffusion is greatly reduced in the body tissues. For the body to increase the rate of diffusion as much as possible, the number of capillaries is increased tremendously. The distance between a cell and a capillary is thus reduced to a great extent. The process is further made faster by having a reducing the distance between the cells and the fluid in the capillaries by having the diameter of the capillaries as small as possible. The substances to be exchanged thus only need to travel a short distance during the exchange.

Surface area

Due to a large number of capillaries in the body, the surface area on which the exchange occurs is highly increased hence faster material exchange between the blood and interstitial fluid. If an estimate is made of the number of capillaries in the body of an adult human being, the number comes to between 10 to 14 million capillaries. Owing to their small size, these capillaries only contain between 5 and seven percentage points of the trial amount of blood in the body.

Blood pressure

The pressure of blood in the capillaries is the lowest when the pressure of the rest of the body is considered. When the arteries branch out into the arterioles, the pressure goes down. When the arterioles further branch out to the capillaries, the pressure of blood is depressed further. The reason for the low blood pressure is that it allows for the movement of material between the blood and interstitial fluid at a faster and more efficient rate than if the blood was moving at a faster rate.

FOUR

The Processes of the Microcirculation of Blood

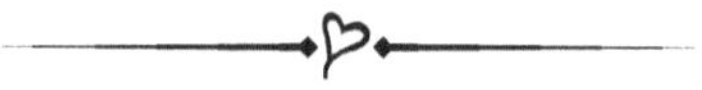

The microcirculation of blood allows the taking the place of three main processes which allow for the exchange of materials between the blood and the interstitial fluid. These processes take place at the same time to allow for the quick movement of materials between the two sides of the capillary walls. These processes are diffusion, bulk flow, and transcytosis. The processes are explained below.

Diffusion

The amount of materials exchanged across the walls of the capillaries through the process of diffusion is the highest when compared to the other two processes. The process of diffusion only works if there is a difference in the level of concentration between two regions. In this case, the two regions being focused on are the blood in the capillaries and the interstitial fluid. Since diffusion works by moving substances from areas where they are highly concentrated in regions where they are lowly concentrated, it allows for the exchange of materials between the blood and the interstitial fluid. The substances vital to the cells such as glucose, amino acids, oxygen and others are more contracted in the blood within the walls of the capillaries than in the interstitial fluid. Diffusion will thus force them to move across the walls of the capillaries from the bloodstream to the interstitial fluid. Similarly, the wastes from the cells such as carbon dioxide and other substances are highly concentrated in the interstitial fluid compared to the bloodstream. Through diffusion, these substances will move across the walls of the capillaries to the bloodstream where they will be carried away from the body tissues. The structure of the endothelium is the main determinant of the permeability of the walls of the capillaries. The endothelial cells may be arranged in three different ways thus leading to the classification of the cells of the endothelium into continuous, discontinuous and fenestrated. The continuous structure allows the least amount of substances to be exchanged between the blood and the interstitial fluid. The discontinuous structure permeates a medium level of exchange of substances between the two sides of the capillary walls while the fenestrated structure permeates the highest amount of substances across the walls of the capillaries. Basically, the higher the level of permeability of the endothelium the higher the amount of substances that will pass across the walls. The other forces that combine with diffusion and depend on the concentration of substances between the two sides of the capillary walls are hydrostatic force and osmosis. The three forces (diffusion, osmosis, and hydrostatic force) are called the Starling forces. They are documented basing on the Starling formula.

Bulk Flow

Hydrostatic force, osmosis, and diffusion all rely on the movement of substances across capillary walls in their dissolved form. However, bulk flow focuses on the movement of large undissolved substances across the walls of the capillaries. Such substances are the ones that are not soluble in lipids and thus have to rely on bulk flow and other similar processes to work. This process is also heavily reliant the capillary walls and their structure which is, in turn, determines their permeability. For a tight endothelial structure such as the continuous endothelium, the level of permeability of the capillary walls is highly reduced thus making it difficult for bulk flow to take place. On the other hand, if the walls of the capillaries are highly perforated as the case is in the discontinuous or fenestrated, the level of permeability of the capillary walls is highly increased thus making it easy for bulk flow to take place. If the substances to be exchanged are not soluble in lipids, the best endothelial structure would be the discontinuous cell structure although the fenestrated one is also good at permeating it. The gaps in the discontinuous cell structure allow the large particles to make the crossing from one side of the capillary wall to the other. One other factor that contributes to the process of bulk flow is the difference in pressure between the interstitium (interstitial space) and the bloodstream. The movement of the substances from the bloodstream to the interstitial space would be as a result of the blood hydrostatic pressure (BHP) and the IFOP (interstitial fluid osmotic pressure). The process that sees to this occurrence is called filtration. When the substances flow from the interstitial fluid to the bloodstream, they use bulk flow. This process, which is the opposite of filtration, is called reabsorption. For reabsorption to take place, there has to be a difference in pressure between the interstitial fluid hydrostatic pressure (IFHP) and the blood colloid pressure (BCOP). Given that there are substances here that can either be filtered or reabsorbed, there has to be a net difference in the types of pressure dealt it with here. The net differences in the forces is called the Net Filtration Pressure shortened as NFP. On one side of the equation are the hydrostatic pressures namely the BHP and the IFHP. The other side of the equation has the osmotic pressures namely the IFOP and BCOP. For filtration to take place, the value of the net filtration equation has to be a positive value. For reabsorption to occur, the value of the net filtration pressure has to be a negative one. Together, the four types of pressure are known as the Starling forces.

Transcytosis

The last of the capillary exchange processes is referred to as transcytosis. It is often also called vesicular transport and takes place to move the very large substances through the endothelial cells in the capillary walls. This process starts by the substances having to move from the interstitial fluid into the bloodstream. When the same substances leave the interstitial fluid, they do so through the process of transcytosis. The substances that move by this method are the ones that cannot dissolve in lipids. They include hormones like insulin which will not dissolve in lipids and move through the other processes like osmosis or diffusion. For the substances to move from a cell to the interstitial fluid through the process of transcytosis, they need to use vesicles either to or from the capillary vessels. These vesicles then leave the cells and either go directly to specific parts of the tissue or merge to with other blood vessels so that their contents mix.

FIVE

MICROCIRCULATION OF BLOOD – WHAT EVERYONE SHOULD KNOW ABOUT

The microcirculation of blood is a process that needs to be taken care of in ways that the conventional methods cannot handle with good results. As a matter of fact, the research that goes into the process of microcirculation focuses on how problems at the microscopic levels of the body can be dealt with with the same effectiveness witnessed in the other parts of the body. The leading company in this field is the Bemer Group which has been focusing on the physical vascular therapy methods for s very long time. To the present, the firm has made it very simple to take care of any problems affecting the process of blood microcirculation that, today, one can do the process on their own without the need for medical assistance from a trained professional.

The Bemer Signal

One major problem that has been noted with the microcirculation of blood has been a lack of vasomotion in some patients. Although many firms have tried to do away with this issue, only Bemer has managed to find a solution that actually shows results. The solution is in the form of the Bemer signal. The Bemer signal forms part of the Bemer Physical Vascular Therapy and is the active ingredient in the therapy. For the signal to work, it is formatted into an electromagnetic field so that it can be transported to the specific area of the body being targeted. For the best results, the Bemer signal is sent through the whole body since it is difficult to find out what specific area of the body is having issues with vasomotion. After the signal is sent to the body, it can be tracked as a Bemer wave. The Institute of Microcirculation has confirmed through empirical evidence that the Bemer signal improved the area of vasomotion.

Vasomotion

The focus on vasomotion is due to the fact it is the main determinant of the effectiveness of the process of microcirculation. Vasomotion refers to the vasodilation and vasoconstriction of the blood vessels of the body. These two processes occur in the vessels just before the capillaries namely the arterioles and the vessels after the capillaries called the venules. Given that the capillaries have no muscles, they do not carry out any vasomotion as they are focused on carrying out the various processes of capillary exchange. If vasomotion does not occur well, the level of pressure in the capillaries will not be the right one to allow for the exchange of substances between the blood and the interstitial fluid. If the pressure is either too high or too low as a result of the lack of adequate vasomotion, the cells will not be given the adequate nutrition and will not perform adequately. On the other hand, the cells produce waste products from their various processes thus need the wastes to be carried away from them. If the cells do not have these wastes removed, they will become poisoned and may thus die. Adequate vasomotion ensures that the cells have all the nutrients they need and the cell remains healthy. If the wastes from the cells are left to fill the interstitial space, they will accumulate to such an extent that they will be a breeding ground for the development of pathogens. One can avoid such a scenario if they have the right rates of vasomotion to make sure that the flow of blood is kept within the required limits of pressure. Bemer has been the only company able to make the best signals that improve the rate of vasomotion through their Bemer signal. The company has made the Bemer signal a reliable way to make improvements in the rates of vasomotion given that it is one of the problems plaguing the elderly in most parts of the world. The Bemer signal underwent a lot of rigorous tests that made sure that, indeed, it works as advertised.

The relationship between Bemer and the Institute of Microcirculation grew out of the work of Doctor Klopp who is in charge of the same institution. He has been on the ground working on the ways to improve the circulation of blood at the microcirculation level. However, given that no diagnosis on this level of the body has not been possible, all his efforts have not been successfully rewarded until he met with the experts at the Bemer Group. Although the Bemer experts had been working on this machine for a while, they did not have the empirical evidence of the workings of their machines. The two parties came together, and the result was the Bemer signal. The Institute of Microcirculation has all the equipment to check in real time the effects of anything that has entered the body and how it works. In this way, the Bemer signal was observed in the body, and it was established that it improved the rate of vasomotion by an impressive 28 percentage points. The results were also replicated in similar cases where the individuals had the Bemer signal introduced into their bodies and the empirical evidence established. To this extent, only the Bemer company has been able to obtain such great results. It is proof that physical vascular therapy indeed works as expected although only a few companies are able to make it work. Bemer is one of them.

Microcirculatory Blood Perfusion

Blood perfusion is the delivery of blood to the specific organ or tissue of the body. At the microcirculation level, blood perfusion is at its most delicate phase as characterized by the fact that the blood vessels involved are very small in size and have very thin walls. For this reasons, anything happening to them will adversely affect their effectiveness in the blood perfusion process thus leading to the poor performance of the cells. With physical vascular therapy, the aim is to improve all the processes that take place at this level of circulation without having to open up the body through surgery and other procedures. The Bemer physical vascular therapy has been proven to be the most effective of all procedures that work on the microcirculation system. Tests have proven that this procedure will improve the rate of blood perfusion by an impressive 29 percentage points. Most of the people who underwent the tests were confirmed to improve with even more percentages than the current value although this was the average. As studies continue, one can only expect that the results are still going to get better by the day.

Venous Return

Physical vascular therapy has also been confirmed to increase the rate of venous return. Venous return refers to the amount of blood that returns to the heart after it has gone through other organs of the body. If the circulation system is effective, the amount of blood returning to the heart should be equal to the amount that leaves the heart. However, most people that experience problems with their circulatory system have been found to have a large disparity between the amount of blood flowing into and out of the heart. When there is a prince with the microcirculation system, a lot of blood will be retained not in the tissues and organs of the body. With too much blood in the organs, the cells will not have enough nutrients coming in and waste being taken away. This will lead to the cultivation of conditions that are rife for pathogens to develop and lead to diseases. In most cases, before the problems in the blood can be observed as outward symptoms, they would have progressed to a significant extent. For this reason, physical vascular therapy as carried out by Bemer has been proven to help in the increase of the venous return of the blood to the heart. Tests carried out the Institute of Microcirculation have proven that it will improve the rate of venous return by 32 percentage points. This value is very impressive and is the highest ever achieved by any method used to improve microcirculation.

Oxygen Utilization

Oxygen utilization is the rate at which the body is able to take up the amount of oxygen in the bloodstream. The process starts in the lungs where blood is filled with oxygen while carbon dioxide is removed from it. The blood is then pumped to the rest of the body where to enters the tissues. It is here that oxygen utilization is taken care of. Through the various processes of capillary exchange, oxygen is removed from the bloodstream and into the interstitial cavity where the cells can access it for use in producing energy. The amount of oxygen removed from the bloodstream to the interstitial fluid is reliant upon the effectiveness of the processes involved in moving the oxygen across the walls of the capillaries. Given that oxygen would be dissolved and is easily moved in the bloodstream, the process that will be used is diffusion. Diffusion relies on the differences in the concentration of molecules in one region compared to the other. With more oxygen molecules in the blood than the interstitial fluid, oxygen will move across the walls of the capillaries to the interstitial cavity. However, diffusion and other processes in involved in the movement of materials across the walls of the capillaries rely on the pressure in the capillaries. For a start, the pressure has to be the lowest possible but not stagnant. Oxygen will thus be utilized only if its concentration in the bloodstream is higher than that in the interstitial fluid. If the blood stays too long, the oxygen will start coming back into the bloodstream, and the cells will not make good use of it. If on the other hand, the blood moves too quickly, the cells will still be starved of oxygen as diffusion will not be allowed to take place effectively. This process will be determined by the effectiveness of the vasomotion of the arterioles and the venules and how they can regulate the pressure of the blood in the capillaries. Given that the Bemer signal has been proven to improve vasomotion, it is only logical that its effect on the rate of oxygen utilization is gauged from the same process. When the amount of blood entering an organ through the arteries is checked and compared to the amount of oxygen in the blood leaving the organ through the veins, it is established that there is an oxygen concentration disparity. This disparity can be used to gauge the level of oxygen utilization. The higher the disparity, the better the oxygen utilization. When the level of oxygen utilization is taken then the physical vascular therapy is applied, there is an increase in the oxygen utilization level by a whole 29 percentage points. That value confirms the effectiveness of the Bemer signal in the improvement of the microcirculation system.

The Future of Healthcare

The circulatory system is one of the most important systems in the body. There are very delicate parts of this system and most of them can to be replaced by simple organ transplants. One can only imagine the cost of a heart transplant given that fact that it is out of the reach of most people today. The circulatory system also poses a problem when it is considered just how delicate it is to make a heart transplant. The heart, being the most important organ in the circulatory system, requires to be both in a healthy condition and compatible with the recipient's body. Such complexities have led to the need to simply take care of the heart rather than seeking treatment after the problem has escalated. Prevention, as they say, always beats cure. The Bemer Group has been dealing with problems of the circulatory system for a long time, and their level of expertise is confirmed through their equipment and methods. Their focus on the microcirculation level has been groundbreaking as evidenced by the equipment they have on the market.

Microcirculation affects the blood pressure in ways that have been confirmed through tests carried out by the Bemer group. Among the problems that are a result of issues in the microcirculation system are hypertension. Hypertension is the case where the body has more blood pressure than the normal parameters. With more people reporting cases of hypertension, is it only normal that firms such as Bemer will have their eyes trained on it. With too much pressure in the blood, the body will have a hard time controlling the main processes in the body. Previous methods of dealing with hypertension were focused on the internal organs such as the heart and the large vessels that carry blood to and from the organs. However, the future is focused on the smaller sections of the body such as the tissues and how they affect the flow of blood in the body. The focus has been placed on the microcirculation system which is the smallest of all the parts of the circulatory system. The Bemer group has proven that microcirculation is the solution to the issues faced by all the other organs of the body in terms of the circulatory system.

SIX

HYPERTENSION AND MICROCIRCULATION

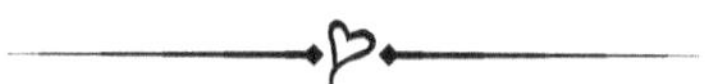

The effects of hypertension on the microcirculation system are undeniable. This process will affect microcirculation in various ways which shall be dealt with in the following sections. The three methods that shall be explained here take place either together or in isolation.

- The first way hypertension affects the microcirculation system is through making the vasomotion processes abnormal such that the rates of vasodilation and vasoconstriction difficult to take place. When the pressure is too much outside the capillaries, the blood arterioles are required to relax or vasodilate so that the pressure is kept constant inside the arterioles. However, hypertension will render the arterioles unable to relax and thus increase the blood pressure in the capillaries. Also, when the pressure outside the capillaries is too low to match that in the capillaries, the arterioles are required to vasoconstrict so that they keep the pressure at the same level in the set parameters.

- The second way hypertension affects the microcirculation system is by changing the structure of the vessels involved in the same system. The vessels are very thin compared to the ones found in the rest of the body. For this reason, they are very sensitive to changes in their structure. Any increase or decrease in the thickness or rigidity of the walls of the vessels will make it difficult for the microcirculation system to takes place effectively. Hypertension increases the ration of the vessels' walls to the lumen. With the increased ratio, the blood flowing them will increase in pressure to an extent where the exchange of substances across the walls of the capillaries will be rendered almost impossible.

- The last way in which hypertension affects the microcirculation system is by causing changes in the density vessels of the body. The microvascular network is the setup of capillaries, arterioles and venules in the body for each organ. Hypertension causes either a reduction (rarefaction) or increase in the density of these vessels. If the density of the vessel increases, the amount of blood pressure will also decrease. This is due to the fact that the high number of branches will reduce the pressure that flows through them. If on the other hand, the density reduces, the level of blood pressure is highly increased. Both cases will make it difficult for the microcirculation system to operate as required.

These methods in which hypertension renders it effects on the microcirculation system have been the method followed by the methods used by antihypertensive therapists in their trials in making it possible to do away with hypertension. The first method employed by these therapists was focused on changing the vasomotion tone and then increasing the rate of vasodilation in the vessels of the body. The therapists then moved their attention to reducing the resistance of the vessels; an occurrence which is a result of the hypertension. Recent studies and methods have been trained on correcting the changes that have been brought about by the differences in the densities of the vessels that take part in the microcirculation system. The issue with these methods has been that most of the agents used in treating this condition have been established to have side effects such as chronic actions. The result sin that they have become complicated and they made it impossible to recommend them.

Pressure in the Bloodstream

The body works by increasing or decreasing the amount of blood pressure in the body to make sure that it remains within the stated parameters. The best scenario is that it should reduce when entering the smaller vessels of the body such as the arterioles and the capillaries and increase when leaving the tissues such as through the venules. What that means is that the pressure of the blood is entering and leaving an organ should be kept the same at all times. However, that is not always the case especially given the fact that there are cases where the body has conditions such as hypertension and other blood circulation problems.

Hypertension and Hydrostatic Pressure

In hypertension, the body experiences various changes which are all deviations from the norm. In normal circumstances, the pressure of the blood leaving the heart stays the same in all areas of the body. When the body is experiencing hypertension, the blood pressure is increasingly made higher as there is a higher level of the peripheral vascular resistance in response to the blood flow. This leads to a significant rise in the total pressure of the blood in the whole body. One part of the body that will experience the highest increase in the pressure of the blood given this condition is the precapillary vasculature. When the level of resistance to the blood has been increased considerably, the amount of pressure in the amount of blood reaching the arteries and arterioles is affected adversely. Very little pressure is made available to the small vessels thus immensely hampering the process of microcirculation.

How Hypertension Brings about and the Abnormalities in Microcirculation

The only way to keep the pressure in the capillaries at a constant level is by having the arterioles and the venules dilate and constrict in response to the pressure of the blood outside the tissues. The problem comes about as a result of having the diameter of the small vessels decrease by a large extent. Due to hypertension, the lumen of the arterioles and venules is significantly reduced. According to physics, a decrease in the size of the lumen will lead to an increase in the pressure of the blood flowing within it. An increase in the ratio between the media and the lumen is the reason why the blood pressures will increase. This case is mostly noted when the body is under a condition that is not permeated to be present. The blood pressure will thus affect the way the microcirculation system works. One case that has been associated with lots of danger is that of hypertension causing an issue in the number of microvessels in the body. When the hypertension reduces the number of microvessels in an organ and tissue, the particular tissue will have poor nourishment and lower ventilation. This issue takes place in stages the first of which makes them vasoconstrict. This occurs due to an increase in the amount of stimuli present and needing them to vasoconstrict. Also, given that hypertension makes the microvessels very sensitive to the vasoconstriction stimuli, it will quick for them to reduce the size of their lumen and thus increase the pressure. When the condition escalates, the process of blood perfusion can be rendered impossible. After this stage, the vessels will keep on constricting until the vessels cannot allow blood to flow through them. With time, they will disappear in totality. What this means is that the person will not be able to have circulation in the part of the tissue which has no more vessels. One way to prove this has been in the case where the fingers of the patients with hypertension will have fewer capillaries than the rest of the body. With time, the fingers will need to have other methods taken care of so that they can blood circulation back on track and the fingers regain their normal functioning. The good bit about this is that the fingers can have better circulation once again using the Bemer signal which has been in use for quite a while now. It will excite the capillaries once more so that they can maintain the normal functioning.

One thing that needs to be observed at all times is the fact that the process of making a diagnosis of hypertension is that some people will experience the same problems in the fingers that can be experienced when one has scleroderma, syndrome X, and hypertrophic cardiomyopathy. One has to combine this case with that of the other symptoms of hypertension to confirm that the individual indeed had hypertension. This test can thus not be used in isolation to confirm a case of hypertension.

Another issue that is brought about by the reduction in the density and the number of the small blood vessels is that the surface area for the exchange of materials between the blood and the interstitial fluid is considerably reduced. When the blood vessels reduce in number and the surface area of capillary exchange reduced, the distance between the cells and the capillaries is also increased significantly. The result is that the cells will have a difficult time accessing the nutrition and having the wastes around them taken away. In general, the result will be that there will be poor performance of the microcirculation system.

The Microcirculation System And How it Increases Hypertension

While hypertension renders the microcirculation system ineffective, there are ways in which the same system contributes to the prevalence of this disease. Studies have pointed out that the relationship between the microcirculation system and hypertension may lead to the increase of the latter and decrease of the former. When the vessels of the microcirculation system note that the pressure of blood in the body has increased for some reason or the other, they respond by limiting the amount of blood that reaches the capillaries. They do so by vasodilation which will in effect reduce the pressure of the blood flowing through them. However, given that hypertension increases the blood pressure to levels which are not safe, the microcirculation system will only serve to increase the level of pressure in the whole body. As the hypertension increases the pressure further, the microcirculation system also limits the level of blood going through them. The result is a vicious circle which the two cases keep on helping one another increase the pressure of the blood in the body. The result will be that the body, rather than protecting itself from harm caused by hypertension, will be aiding hypertension to grow by leaps and bounds. The problem is that the body will be acting naturally to keep the pressure of the blood within the tissues within the set parameters.

One way to prove this relationship was from a study carried out by a group of scientists on the relationship between the weight of a baby at birth and the weight of the placenta. While the two may seem like pieces that have little relations with each other, the results were surprising. When the relationship was inverse such that the baby was born small, but the placenta was a big one, the individual would grow up with a high likelihood of having bad pressure when adults. This means that a small baby with a large placenta will likely have high blood pressure. The inverse, which had large babies with small weights for the placenta, found out that the babies were less likely to have high blood pressure when they grew up. The researchers gave an explanation that has been proven in other tests of a similar kind. They stated that when the placenta was large in relation to the baby, the amount of blood the flowed to their trunk was limited. For this reason, the baby would have a poorly developed microcirculation system when they grew up. This issue would be accompanied by the likely occurrence of hypertension if the baby grew up to be an adult. The same researchers came to the conclusion that the poor development of the microcirculation system also lead to the likely development of anomalies in the circulatory system of the baby when they grew into adults. It has been demonstrated before that the occurrence of a poorly developed microcirculation system will lead to the presence of pathogens or other problems of the circulatory system. With the equivalent from Bemer, one can have the child undergo certain procedures which will help them get rid of the problems as they grow up.

Microcirculation and the Prevention of Damage to End-Organs

With the correct administration and care, some of the methods employed by antihypertensive therapists have been proven to prevent and even reduce the prevalence of certain problems of the circulatory system like stroke and coronary heart disease. The problem comes in when it is confirmed that most of the diseases of this nature cause end-organ damage and they include nephropathy, retinopathy, lacunar infarction, microvascular angina and others. The problem is further escalated by the fact that these issues have a close relationship with the microcirculation system and hypertension. With technologies from The Bemer Group, patients have been helped to do away with the issues of preventing hypertension and similar issues. Better yet, given that these ailments have been known to cause end-organ damage, one can save their bodies using Bemer techniques and approaches.

- **Microalbuminuria**

Microalbuminuria is also known as the case of increased excretion of albumin. This case has been among the main risk factors for most cardiovascular diseases in people who are either suffering from diabetes or not. Some studies have confirmed that those with hypertension have higher chances of having proteinuria cases when compared to their counterparts without hypertension. If one has hypertension, they up to three times more likely to have proteinuria than the individuals who do not have the same issue. While the case of having microalbuminuria is a reversible one, there needs to be a lot more care when handling it than other cases of the circulatory system. The best to deal with such a vase would be making sure that the person does not skip their allocated medical procedures as noted in the case of the methods and physical vascular therapy from the likes of Bemer and other firms. Bemer stands out from the crowd for this effectiveness since it has the best machines and methods of doing way with such procedures.

· Microcirculation in the Myocardium

The heart is the most resilient of all the organs of the body. When an individual dies, it is among the last organs to also die out. It also starts working very early in the life of the person and will not stop until they are dead. This structure would printout to a very effective organ that will not die out easily. However, it can also be a victim of end organ damage if it incurs changes in the structures of the small vessels that supply its muscles with food and oxygen and take away wastes and carbon dioxide. This problem can be developed either in adulthood due to diseases such as hypertension or early in life. In the latter scenario, the fetus will have a poorly developed set of myocardial microvessels. As the fetus grows up and becomes an adult, it will have a significantly higher chance of suffering from end-organ damage.

· Cerebral Microcirculation

A person suffering from hypertension is very likely to suffer from stroke given the nature of their disease. Lacunar infarction, which is the presence of tiny but deep infarcts that occur after the rupture of veins in the body, has been cited as one of the main reason why people suffer from stroke and other similar cases of the circulatory system. Hypertension will cause many different changes in the structure of the cerebral arterioles which can be observed in the increase in the ratio of the media to lumen ratio. Also, the die matter of the vessels will be highly rescued hence increasing the pressure of the blood flowing through them. This increased pressure will increase the likelihood of their rupturing under the heavy toll and lead to stroke. One can only be happy that the presence of the condition of hypertension does not lead to the rarefaction of the cerebral arterioles and the capillaries of the brain. If that were the case, the rates of stroke would be heightened by a large extent and the people with hypertension would have a higher likelihood of suffering from a stroke. Even better is the fact that some of the methods used in antihypertensive therapy have been proved to reverse the undesirable changes brought about in the structure of the microvessels in the cerebral circulatory system. This significantly reduces the chances of having a stroke even for patients with hypertension. Given that the Bemer signal does work better than most of these issues, it will be the best approach to be used for this case.

SEVEN

Treating of Hypertension in the Microcirculatory System

---❥---

When on is targeting parts of the microcirculation system when treating hypertension while also aiming to prevent end-organ damage, their focus should be on the reduction of the ration between the walls and the lumen of the vessels. They should also focus on finding out ways to reverse the process of microvascular rarefaction. There are many ways to do so, and all of them are considered to be antihypertensive agents. They include;

Beta-Blockers (β-Blockers)

These agents have not proven to possess any significant effects in the restoring of the structural changes that would have occurred in the small vessels of an individual's body. Some of the most used beta-blockers on the market are propranolol and atenolol both of which have poor records in the treatment of the effects of hypertension on a person's microcirculatory system.

Diurectics

Diuretics include using compounds and methods such as hydrochlorothiazide therapy which have proven to be of very little effectiveness in their trial to restore the structure of the vessels that take part in microcirculation.

Alpha-Blockers (α-Blockers)

The alpha-blockers have displayed some quite promising results when it comes to tests carried out in experimental situations. The α-adrenoreceptor blockade agents such as prazosin have proven to increase the density in the capillaries within the tissues in the body.

ACE Inhibitors

ACE inhibitors have had mixed results although the general trend has been a positive one so far. Their main role has been the reduction in the ratio of the media to the lumen of the vessels involved in microcirculation thus making it possible to increase the level of microcirculation. Their main issue has been that the very same ACE inhibitors tend to change the structure of the venules and arterioles of the body. They do so by reducing their densities. As explained before, lower densities lead to a poor response to the stimuli needed to initiate either vasodilation or vasoconstriction. One thus not bank on the ACE inhibitors as they need further studies to establish their worth and level of effectiveness. Otherwise, they will remain in test format.

Calcium Antagonists

These types of agents have proven their worth in restoring the structure of the vessels that are involved in the process of microcirculation. Among the variants available in this group are nimodipine, verapamil, and nifedipine which have given a lot of hope to those who want to use them.

Combination therapy

When each of the methods above has given differing results, the aim has been to combine other methods and to lean on their ability to provide effective results for the whole process. So far, the methods have been very effective to the point where they are deemed to be the best solution or this case. One can combine beta-blockers with ACE inhibitors to get results which are better than when only a single method is applied on its own. When an ACE inhibitor such as perindopril is combined with diuretic indapamide, the results have been the increase in the density and diameter of the capillaries of the body. Both results are desirable and have been in use for a while now.

EIGHT

THE BEMER GROUP

The Bemer Group has been offering some of the best treatment equipment in the alleviation of issues that plague the microcirculation system. The group has been operating for a long time now. The quality of its work has been seen by its being in possession of some very prestigious documentations such as an ISO 13485 certification together with a reddot design award for the year 2013. It has also made a reputation for itself due to being one of the leading providers of physical vascular therapy and other similar methods all of which are geared towards the support of the body in its efforts to healing itself as far as restoring its natural structure of the various vessels that carry out the microcirculation system.

This group will put one in the possession of medical personnel that is highly qualified in dealing with the health issues they have. The methods used by the Bemer group are under the protection of patents as they are the results of high levels of research that has gone on for a very long time. The company is including the latest findings as far as the field of microcirculation is concerned with the methods and equipment being used. These methods ensure that all of its patients and clients get the very best of healthcare from this company.

The Products from the Bemer Group

This great company offers just two main product types namely The Classic Set and The BEMER Pro Set. In addition to that, the firm has many application modules like the comfort chair (B.COMFORT), Small-Scale treatment (B.PAD), Light Treatment (B.LIGHT), Selective treatment (B.SPOT), Full Body treatment (B.BODY Pro), Seat cushion (B.SIT) and its Full Body treatment (B.BODY Classic). All the application modules are put together with other accessories to make that each of the machines listed above are in great working conditions and give the very best of results for the tests and treatments carried out. The set of accessories includes Handle (B.GRIP), Wall mounting, Fixing strap, signal tester (B.SCAN), foot protection, power supply unit, protection glasses, car power cable, the rechargeable battery which powers each of the machines just in the case the power is not available as needed.

The BEMER Pro Set

This machine is the very best of an all-in-one remedy for the procedure of Physical Vascular Therapy since it has each and every tool that one may be in need of when carrying out the procedures of physical vascular therapy. Looking at this machine, one would conclude that The Bemer Group and its reddot design award come out clearly in this design and ergonomics of this machine. It comes with a touch screen which has easily-usable items that are clearly in arrangement making it easy to see the various options they will need in selecting to effect their treatments. With a simple touch of the finger, the patient can easily start their own treatment with guaranteed best results in using the machine. The machine lacks any signals or commands on its touchscreen display. Each of the commands on its touchscreen easily guides the user through the various treatment steps that can be easily performed. The great part is that this display can be easily used in controlling two machines at a single time when the user turns on the 2-in-1 mode which has proven to be very useful. There is no need in obtaining a control panel for each machine with this control. The machine also features many application modules and accessories that make it the best for use in providing physical vascular therapy. This BEMER Pro Set goes to work through the use application modules that are vital in conducting the BEMER signal that is generated in its control unit. This control unit allows for treating the exact parts of the body that need this treatment.

Other than the normal and standardized treatment procedures that can be applied according to one's needs, the BEMER Pro Set also has three pre-set programs that work through the facilitation of intensively treating the specific areas affected. One can select the areas for treatment from the B.BOX control unit that has ten intensity levels for the user to make a choice from. This BEMER Pro Set comes with other capabilities and functions.

The BEMER Classic Set

This Classic Set from Bemer is meant for the users who are only starting out with the idea of physical vascular treatment in their programs. The set comes with lots of benefits such easily usable user interface on its graphic display, the ability to use three steps in the program for flexibility in use, ten varying levels of the intensity of treatment, and a regeneration and sleep program that allows the recovery of the body from each treatment session. One can obtain the whole set directly from the online platform of the company.

NINE

CONCLUSION

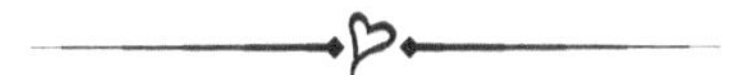

The system of microcirculation has a very vital role in the normal functioning of the human body. By this process, one's body tissues obtain oxygen and nutrients that are delivered to tissues for it to function properly. Also, this very system makes sure that all the wastes from the cell activities are removed to eliminate any chances of pathogens or the death of the tissues and organs. This microcirculation system is the one that keeps the blood pressure in the organs and tissues at a constant level using vasomotion processes such as vasoconstriction and vasodilation of the vessels' walls.